MW00945204

Eczema No More

The Complete Guide to Natural Cures
for Eczema; and a Holistic System to
End Eczema & Clear Your Skin
Naturally & Permanently

Jason S. Bradford

Copyright© 2014 by Jason S. Bradford

Eczema No More

Copyright© 2014 Jason S. Bradford

All Rights Reserved.
Warning: The unauthorized reproduction or distribution of this copyrighted work is illegal. No part of this book may be scanned, uploaded or distributed via internet or other means, electronic or print without the author's permission. Criminal copyright infringement without monetary gain is investigated by the FBI and is punishable by up to 5 years in federal prison and a fine of $250,000. (http://www.fbi.gov/ipr/). Please purchase only authorized electronic or print editions and do not participate in or encourage the electronic piracy of copyrighted material.

Publisher: Living Plus Healthy Publishing

ISBN-13: 978-1500328467

ISBN-10: 1500328464

Disclaimer

The Publisher has strived to be as accurate and complete as possible in the creation of this book. While all attempts have been made to verify information provided in this publication, the Publisher assumes no responsibility for errors, omissions, or contrary interpretation of the subject matter herein. Any perceived slights of specific persons, peoples, or organizations are unintentional.

This book is not intended for use as a source of legal, business, accounting or financial advice. All readers are advised to seek services of competent professionals in the legal, business, accounting, and finance fields.

The information in this book is not intended or implied to be a substitute for professional medical advice, diagnosis or treatment. All content contained in this book is for general information purposes only. Always consult your healthcare provider before carrying on any health program.

Table of Contents

Introduction

Eczema, also called atopic dermatitis, is probably the most common skin disease. There are several variants to the disease, such as contact dermatitis, caused by contact with an allergen, dyshydrotic eczema, caused by exposure to water and seborrheic dermatitis, caused by oils in the skin. Eczema can affect everyone from babies to old people. Fifteen million people will suffer from eczema at some time in their lives and ten percent of them are infants or young children.

Eczema is like an allergy; in effect, it is a hypersensitivity reaction to some type of allergen. Some researcher surmise that those who suffer from eczema are missing essential proteins that, when absent, make the skin more sensitive.

Eczema is related to people who have asthma and seasonal allergies. People who get eczema often have a family history of this condition as well as of asthma and seasonal allergies.

Things that relate to getting eczema include the following:

- Flu
- Colds
- Dry winter air
- Allergies to just about anything
- Stressful emotions
- Excessive exposure to water
- Irritant or chemical exposure
- Temperature fluctuations
- Dyes or fragrances to beauty products

What are some common symptoms you might have with eczema? The skin may be dry or bumpy, especially on the backs of the arms and the fronts of the thighs. Blisters can show up that ooze and crust over. There can be itchiness of the skin along with redness or thick areas of the skin after having the condition for a long time.

Eczema involves different body areas. In kids under the age of 2, the rash of eczema is seen on the scalp, the face, the hands and the feet. In older kids and adults, common areas of eczema include the inside aspect of the knees and elbows. Severe outbreaks can involve rashes anyplace on the body.

Doctors can usually tell whether or not you have eczema just by looking at your skin and by asking you about your personal and family history. Sometimes allergy skin testing is necessary to make sure you really have eczema. In cases where your eczema is difficult to treat or when you have other allergic symptoms along with skin rashes, doctors often check for skin allergies.

There are many treatments for eczema, which will be discussed in this guide. For those with no medical or natural therapies available, it may be good enough to moisturize the skin and to avoid scratching the affected skin. Fortunately, there are medications you will learn about that take care of the itch when you absolutely can't stand it. You can even make sure your child's fingernails are cut short so they don't damage the skin with itching.

There are also things you can do to avoid getting eczema. These include giving eggs and other allergic foods to young children, staying away from lanolin and wool, using milder soaps that don't contain a lot of chemicals or solvents and avoiding changes in temperature.

Keeping a low stress level helps as well as avoiding triggers that you know cause you to have excessive symptoms.

You should minimize contact with water and use body washes or cleansers instead of harsh soaps. The bathwater should be as cool as you can tolerate as long, hot baths can make things worse. Avoid heavy scrubbing of the skin and make strong use of ointments, lotions or creams to soften the skin immediately after bathing. Ointments and creams contain no alcohol so they tend to be better than lotions.

Eczema has a long-standing prognosis. What this means is that, once you get it, you tend to get it for a very long time. It tends to clear around age 5-6 years of age if you get it as an infant; however, there are commonly flare ups over time. You are more likely to have difficult-to-treat eczema if you have it at a young age, if it occurs with other allergy and asthma symptoms, if a large body area is covered with the disease or if eczema runs strongly in your family.

Complications of eczema will be discussed later in this guide; however, the most common complications include skin infections from openings to the skin and permanent scars, mostly by scratching the skin too much.

While many people can't do anything to prevent eczema, you can prevent it in infants by breastfeeding the infant until they are at least 4 months old. Formulas containing partially hydrolyzed proteins will also protect babies from getting eczema.

In the next chapter, we'll take a serious look at what eczema really is and how you can know if the rash you have is, in fact eczema.

Chapter 1: A Close Look at Eczema

Eczema, also called atopic dermatitis, is a skin rash involving the epidermis of the skin. It actually makes up a wide range of related skin rashes. Its appearance often depends on the location on the body and the age of the individual who has it.

The main signs are redness to the skin, skin tissue swelling, severe itching, dry skin, flaky skin, blisters, crusty skin and areas of oozing of tissue fluid and bleeding from scratching. If a person has chronic disease, there are areas of scars from prior scratches that intermingle between areas of active disease. The word comes from the Greek word "to boil over". This is because of the boils people get when the disease is active.

There are a lot of synonyms for eczema, which makes its diagnosis difficult. For example, you can define eczema on the hand as being "hand eczema" or eczema of the face as being "facial eczema". You can describe eczema that comes in small circles as being "discoid eczema". "Diffuse eczema" occurs in bigger areas of the body. Some patients and doctors call all eczema "atopic dermatitis", which further confuses the picture.

Categories of Eczema

Academic sources have classified "eczema" into different categories that make it somewhat easier to know what you've got. These are the main categories of eczema:

- **Atopic Dermatitis**. This includes the type seen in infants and the type seen in the flexural surfaces of the legs and arms. It is considered both an allergic and hereditary disease, related to those who have hay fever and asthma. It is a very itchy rash occurring in many areas of the body due to exposure to an allergen. It is usually an allergen that is taken into the body as opposed to an allergen that is put on the body externally. It is more common in developed companies than it is in undeveloped countries for reasons that are unclear.

- **Contact Dermatitis**. This can be of the allergic type or the irritant type. If it is due to the allergic type, it means the person has come in contact with an allergen like that found in poison ivy or a nickel allergy. If it is due to an irritant, it usually something like a detergent. The component in detergent called sodium lauryl sulfate is a common cause of irritant dermatitis. Some types of irritant dermatitis is only triggered by the sun and is called phototoxic dermatitis. Fortunately for most cases of contact dermatitis, if one is removed from the allergen or irritant, the rash eventually disappears.

- **Xerotic Eczema**. Some call this the "winter itch" and doctors sometimes call this "pruritis hiemalis". This is seriously dry skin that becomes so dry that it becomes flaky, irritated, itchy and red. It is commonly worse in the winter season and is seen mostly in the trunk and the limbs. The skin becomes tender from frequent itching and there are excoriations from scratching so much. It is seen more often in older people than it is in younger people.

- **Seborrheic Dermatitis**. Commonly called "cradle cap" when seen in newborn infants, it looks a great deal like dandruff in infants. The scales are greasy and peel off with the combing of the hair and scalp. It is fortunately a harmless condition; however, it is unsightly with yellow crusty scalp patches that are difficult to get rid up. Babies eventually outgrow it.

- **Dyshidrotic Eczema**. This can occur on any part of the body but is commonly seen on the palms of the hands and soles of the feet, including the sides of the toes. There are tiny, fluid-filled bumps called vesicles as part of the rash, along with cracks in the skin. It is related to over exposure to water and is worse during warmer weather.

- **Discoid Eczema**. This is also called nummular eczema and involves small, penny-sized areas of skin redness, scaling and inflammation. The rash can be dry or oozing, and has clear boundaries. It is seen much more commonly in dry winter weather and is usually seen on the lower aspects of the legs. It is usually a transient rash of no known cause.

- **Venous Eczema**. This is also called "stasis dermatitis" and occurs when you have increased swelling and varicose veins in your lower extremities. This is more common in people who are older than 50 years of age. The skin is purplish, scaly and itchy and can lead to the development of leg ulcers.

- **Dermatitis Herpetiformis**. Some doctors refer to this as "Duhring's disease". It is an incredibly itchy skin disease found on the back, arms, legs and knees. It is related to also having celiac disease of the intestines. Surprisingly, a diet appropriate for those with celiac disease can help reduce the incidence of the rash. Nighttime makes the itching worse.

- **Neurodermatitis**. This is a dermatitis caused by itching the same area over and over again. The skin becomes pigmented and thicker; the itching feeds back on itself and you continue to have itching once the condition takes hold. It is also called lichen simplex chronicus. When you teach yourself to get over the itching and take anti-inflammatory medication, the itching stops and the rash eventually goes away.

- **Autosensitization Eczema**. This is a skin rash that you get when you are infected somewhere on your body with parasites, bacteria, viruses or fungi. Once the infection clears up with medication or your immune system, the rash tends to disappear along with the infection. Interestingly, it always seems to show up a distance away from the site of the infection.

Why We Get Eczema

No one knows exactly how and why we get eczema but doctors and researchers suspect that both genetics and environment have something to do with it. It clearly runs in some families and is more common in industrialized countries.

There is a "hygiene hypothesis" that states that allergic diseases like eczema are more common in cleaner environments. You need, apparently, to be exposed to some bacteria and other immune modulators during our young childhood and, if the environment is too clean, you don't get that.

Some suggest that eczema is related to an allergy to house dust mites. About 5 percent of all people are allergic to dust mite excrement. Even so, it's not completely clear that this is the cause of all eczema.

Interestingly, eczema occurs three times more commonly in those who also have celiac disease and twice as likely as those who have relatives with celiac disease, which could mean that there is some kind of genetic connection between celiac disease and eczema.

How Do You Know It's Eczema?

There is no blood test for eczema and most people get diagnosed by a physician familiar with the look and feel of the disease. In unusual cases, the doctor may need to do a skin biopsy, which can diagnose the presence of eczema.

Skin biopsies involve numbing the skin with xylocaine and taking a small punch out of the skin that extends through all layers of the skin. The skin punch can be as small as 2 mm in diameter. This sample is kept in formalin until a pathologist can look at the samples stained on a slide under a microscope.

Because eczema can have many different appearances, the diagnosis can be difficult to obtain and a biopsy may be the only thing that distinguishes eczema from other skin rashes.

Chapter 2: How Eczema May Affect You

Eczema is usually a chronic disease that has no complications. There can be complications, however, if the affected person itches the rash too much or rash becomes open and infected. The most common complications of eczema include:

- **Neurodermatitis.** This is when itching feeds back on itself so that you get more and more itching. The skin thickens and becomes more leathery. The skin can become darker, more pigmented or redder than your regular skin and permanent scars are a common phenomenon of having scratched too much. Neurodermatitis is a "nerve-related" disease because your nervous itching makes the rash worse than it otherwise would be.

- **Infection of the skin**. This can occur when the scratching opens up a break in the skin or when dry patches make fissures in the skin that allow bacteria to inoculate themselves, causing an infection. This process is called impetiginization because the end result is "impetigo" or skin bacterial infections. The most likely organism to cause such an infection is Staphylococcus aureus. The treatment is warm packs and sometimes antibiotics to kill the infection.

- **Eye complications**. Some people with eczema develop complications affecting their eyes that can, unfortunately, lead to permanent eye damage. The itching around the eyes is usually very severe and the eye waters continually. You also get eye inflammation, a condition called blepharitis, and conjunctivitis, which is an inflammation of the lining of the eyelid. As this is a condition that can lead to permanent eye injury, you should see your doctor or an ophthalmologist for immediate treatment.

- **Eczema herpeticum**. This is a herpes virus infection that happens when the skin becomes infected with cold sores due to a break in the skin and reduced immunity. This can be a serious condition that is very painful. There are groups of blisters that appear in the areas overlying the eczema. The blisters break open and the affected individual can suffer from malaise and a high fever. If you get these symptoms, you should see a doctor right away so antiviral treatment can be started.

- **Psychological distress**. You can suffer from embarrassment and other psychological effects from having eczema. Kids with eczema have more behavioral issues when compared to kids without eczema. These are children who have more dependency on their parents than other kids. Some of these kids need psychological counseling so they can cope with their disease and learn some better ways to be with eczema.

- **Bullying**. Kids with eczema can be victims of bullying in school because of their condition. This bullying can be very traumatic and may result in a child that is quieter than they should be and more withdrawn. For this reason, there are support groups for kids with eczema that can help them deal with their disease better and to find other kids who have the disease that can help them get through without bullying or other inter-relational problems.

- **Sleep problems**. Kids and adults alike have problems sleeping with eczema and the lack of sleep can affect mood and behavior. Most of the time it is the itching that keeps people up but it can be from other complications. Kids can have trouble concentrating at school and adults can have trouble concentrating at work. If you have a child with eczema, it makes sense to let the teacher know so that if the child gets behind in their work, the teacher can at least know the reason.

- **Self-confidence issues**. Those who suffer from atopic eczema often lack self-confidence, whether they are adults or children. Kids can suffer from problems with a poor image and this can affect their social skills and development. These kids need a great deal of support and encouragement so that they don't suffer from poor self-esteem on a chronic basis. See a therapist or counselor if self-confidence issues seem to be a problem, whether the person having the problem is an adult or a child.

Chapter 3: Traditional Treatments for Eczema

There is no real cure for eczema. Fortunately, some people outgrow the condition or they have a spontaneous remission. Others can manage on conventional medical therapy, which is aimed at controlling the itching and inflammation of the disease and at making the person with eczema feel better. Conventional medical treatment can help people with eczema function in life with a minimum of discomfort.

Moisturizers are some of the best therapy for eczema. Therapies like Aquaphor® and Eucerin® used especially after a bath can trap moisture in the skin and are safe to use at any age. Using lotions, on the other hand, can be a bad thing because lotions almost always contain some type of alcohol, which can be drying to the skin, especially skin afflicted with eczema. One good cheap treatment is to use Petrolatum Jelly just after a lukewarm bath and while the affected area is still wet.

Commonly used medication for eczema is corticosteroid cream. It can be found over the counter and decreases the inflammation in the skin. You can get low potency, medium potency and high potency creams. Low potency creams are reserved for infants with eczema and with other mild forms of the disease. The medium and high potency creams need a prescription from the doctor but are better for severe cases of the disease.

Medications that control itching will also help reduce the discomfort of the disease and therefore its appearance and the presence of scarring. There are topical antihistamines in the form of Benadryl® Cream or oral antihistamines. Sometimes it is better to use the sedative forms of antihistamines because they help you relax and feel less itchy. Some of the sedative antihistamines include hydroxyzine (Atarax®) and diphenhydramine (Benadryl®). Both are very effective in reducing itching but both make you very tired.

In certain cases, taking prednisone for a brief period of time can help control the inflammation and appearance of eczema. It should only be used in short term experiences because of the negative side effects of prednisone or corticosteroid dependence.

Severe cases of eczema can be treated through the use of oral immunosuppressant drugs such as cyclosporine (Neoral®, Sandimmune®) and methotrexate. These may be necessary if the less strong medications seem not to have the desired effect on the eczema. Another drastic therapy involves the use of medications that sensitize the skin to light and the use of ultraviolet therapy. Again, this therapy is used only when no other treatment seems to work.

There are two creams recently approved by the FDA for the management of eczema. The first is called Protopic® or tacrolimus and Elidel® or pimecrolimus. These are cacineurin inhibitors that work in people who have eczema and are at least 2 years old. The goal is to block the immune system hyperactivity that seems to be present in those who have the disease. There is a black box warning on the use of these creams because it isn't known if there are any long term complications of taking these medications. Because they block the immune system, they shouldn't be used in any situation where the individual already has an immune deficiency problem and who might develop infections or cancer because of low immune system activity. Some people have gotten cancer from taking these anti-immune system drugs.

Antibiotics may be necessary for the treatment of eczema that has gotten infected due to itching or cracking of the skin. These tend to be used for short time periods and only when an infection is likely to be present. Your doctor will need to prescribe antibiotics in cases of cellulitis complicating eczema.

Allergy shots have been tried for eczema but have not been proven very helpful. This is because there is no identifiable allergen associated with this condition.

Conventional therapies for eczema tend to work on most people who try them; however, they have a number of side effects that make it difficult to use these forms of therapy. Antihistamines can cause extreme exhaustion and fatigue; corticosteroid cream can contribute to infections of the skin and immunosuppressants can cause infections and some cancers.

There are fortunately, dietary and other remedies that you can use for the treatment of eczema that are relatively free of side effects and are just as potent and helpful for eczema as are the expensive conventional treatments.

As always, you should see your doctor if you have a worrisome rash but should also read about your condition so that you know about natural treatments that really work!

Chapter 4: Treating Eczema with Diet and Lifestyle Changes

Foods have the potential to cure or cause eczema and there are things you can do in your lifestyle that can control symptoms without drugs or medications. It is important to see if you are allergic to any of the foods that commonly cause eczema. In such cases, your eczema could be cured just by switching out a specific food or two that unknowingly exacerbates your symptoms.

One of the most common allergy-producing foods is wheat or wheat products. You can find wheat in cakes, cookies, wheat-based breads, crackers, pretzels, many snack foods, gravy, pasta and soy sauce. It often takes very little of wheat intake to provoke an allergic response that shows up as wheat allergies.

Gluten is a component of wheat that can be the ultimate cause of wheat allergies. Unfortunately, gluten can also be found in barley, oats and rye. Gluten allergies often cause gastrointestinal symptoms, too, such as stomach upset and chronic diarrhea. If you have these symptoms along with eczema, it is likely that gluten and wheat likely have something to do with it. Stop the wheat and gluten products and your skin may likely clear up.

Dairy products are also common contributors to the cause of eczema. Dairy products don't just mean milk. The following products are considered dairy products: cottage cheese, ice cream, yogurt and cheese. Unfortunately, dairy products can be hidden in a number of desserts, including baked goods and other recipes.

What are some other foods that could be the source of your eczema? Think about these foods:

- Eggs
- Seafood
- Nuts
- Corn
- Soy products
- Citrus foods
- Highly acidic foods
- Honey
- Certain spices

- Caffeine
- Salty foods
- Chocolate
- Highly processed foods

The trick with knowing which foods are causing the eczema is doing a food diary that is enmeshed with a symptom diary. When you think you may have the offending agent, go ahead and eliminate it from your diet for up to two weeks and see how your eczema does. If it gets better, the food might be the cause of the eczema and you should continue avoiding it.

Babies can get eczema from drinking cow's milk-based formulas or even from drinking soy-based formulas. Fortunately, eczema is very rare in breastfed babies. For this reason alone, babies should be breastfed as long as possible. Formula companies also make "elemental formulas" that are made of proteins that have been broken down. These usually do not cause allergies or eczema but are terrible tasting.

Sometimes, breastfed babies can be allergic to something in mom's diet. It may be that mom has to go through an elimination diet challenge to see what is bothering her baby.

The trick is to find alternatives to foods that make you itch and substitute those in your diet. If it's wheat that causes your eczema, eat only gluten-free foods. Read labels and eat foods that don't make you feel like you're food deprived. The lack of itching should be motivation enough to keep you from eating foods that make your eczema worse.

Elimination diets usually work but you should do this under the care of a physician or nurse practitioner who can make sure that you have the proper nutrition while you are undergoing this challenge. They can also help you identify which foods are the trigger as sometimes the connection isn't noticed until the food is added back to the diet and the itching flares up.

Using Your Body's Natural Cycle

First of all, make sure that the meat, grains and produce you eat is organically grown. This is food that is absent of pesticides and certain herbicides that can make the foods prone to causing eczema even though it isn't the food itself.

There is a lot to be said about the natural body metabolism cycle—a twenty four hour cycle that, if followed, can decrease the rate of eczema symptoms. There are three different metabolic periods you need to consider:

1. **Elimination and maintenance**: This is a period from about 4 am to noon and is when the cells are getting rid of their waste products, manufacturing cells and repairing damaged cells. There are foods you need to eat at breakfast that promote these bodily activities.

2. **Digestion**: This happens between noon and 8:00 pm. This when most of our digestion takes place and should be when most of the food in our body is ingested. The earlier you eat this "biggest meal of the day", the better off you are.

3. **Assimilation**: This is when the body mobilizes the nutrients you have eaten and brings them to the cells to participate in cellular functions. This period of the day begins at 8:00 pm and ends at about 4:00 pm. You generally aren't supposed to eat much during this time.

So how do you eat in ways that are the most compliant with these metabolic phases your body is going through? You basically start with breakfast. Breakfast should be started with plenty of fruits. Raw fruits are better than cooked fruits. Make sure you eat the skins if possible. You can easily make a fruit smoothie with coconut water, your favorite fruits and a blender.

Select fruits with the lowest glycemic index possible. This means that the fruit has enough fiber in it to keep the sugar-part of the food from flowing quickly into the bloodstream. The best fruits to choose from are oranges, cherries, apples, peaches, berries, pears and plums.

Add ground golden flaxseeds to the smoothie for better fiber and think about adding blue green algae, green drink mix, probiotics and organic coconut oil. This makes a super food drink that's great for helping your body do what it needs to during its first metabolic phase.

Lunchtime should definitely be eaten before 4:00 in the afternoon. This should be the biggest meal of your day and should be cooked or served with unheated coconut oil or extra virgin olive oil. The vegetables you choose should be steamed slightly in a steamer or served raw. You should pair your vegetables with any one of the following choices: halibut, salmon, oysters, sweet potatoes, brown rice, potatoes, goat cheese, boiled eggs or sprouted grains bread. You can also have things like Miso soup with vegetables, salads, sautéed mushrooms with salad and mashed potatoes cooked with coconut milk and butter.

Dinner occurs during the digestion period so you should have it and finish it by 8:00 pm. The thing you definitely need to include in this meal is a glass of vegetable juice. Vegetable juice can clear up eczema easily. The drink should be a large one, consisting of 16 to 24 ounces of dark green vegetable juice that includes kale, parsley, zucchini, cucumber, green bell pepper, celery or cilantro. A mixture of these vegetables is definitely best.

Other vegetables to include:

- Two stalks of celery—these have a basic diuretic effect and helps eliminate carbon dioxide from the body. Acidic foods can be counteracted by eating this vegetable.

- Parsley—half a bunch. This cleanses the body of toxins and aids in the function of various bodily functions. It is also high in nutrients.

- Carrots—two medium ones. Try not to cut off the top because it contains the most phytonutrients in the vegetable. You can discard the green shoots but leave the very top on when you blend it.

- Cilantro—1/4 bunch. Cilantro has the ability to get rid of heavy metals in the body, including lead, cadmium and mercury.

- Kale—two to three leaves. There are a lot of nutrients in kale, which is known for its cancer-fighting properties. It is very high in carotenoids that fight cancer and it also has a lot of easily-absorbable calcium in it so that disorders of bone loss and skin diseases can be helped by eating kale.

- Cucumber—1/2 cucumber. This has diuretic properties that remove fluids from the body. It cleanses the blood from toxins.

- Apple—one cut-up apple. This is basically used to sweeten the juice and to make it more palatable.

Some additions to the basic juice include a quarter of a beet, some cabbage leaves, zucchini, bok choy and bell pepper.

If you drink the above drink and you still feel hungry, raw nuts and raw seeds can fill you up. They should be organic if at all possible. Some choices include pumpkin seeds, sunflower seeds, soaked almonds, pine nuts and walnuts.

So what's good for snacks? You may be too tired to juice up a vegetable juice some nights so you should have a salad mixed with raw nuts. Any types of fruits, fresh or dried, make good snacks for eczema. You can eat cut up pieces of various kinds of vegetables or eat a handful of seeds or nuts that are unsalted.

Lifestyle Management for Eczema

As unfortunate as it is, it's a fact of life that eczema will affect your life. Besides medications, natural remedies, and an eczema diet, there are things you need to do regarding your lifestyle to change what you can about your condition.

The first thing you need to do is reduce skin irritation through lifestyle changes:

- Don't scratch or rub the skin. Scratching or rubbing causes the sensation of itching to feed back on itself so that the itching increases. This is why you need to apply moisturizer whenever you can, especially when you have just washed your hands or body. The moisturizer seals in what moisture your skin has taken in and keeps the skin hydrated.

- Do not wear clothing that has just been purchased without washing it first. New clothing contains irritating chemicals and formaldehyde that fortunately washes out in the washing machine. To make sure the chemicals are out, do a second rinsing of the clothing to get both chemicals and soap out of your clothes.

- Use mild allergy-free laundry soap whenever possible. It contains no dyes or perfumes that can cause skin reactions. The detergent should be clear in color and have no fragrance.

- Wear clothing that is loose weave, like cotton or a cotton blend that allows the skin to breathe and allows air to pass through to the skin. This tends to be more comfortable to wear. Also, avoid wearing anything that is made from wool as this is really irritating, even to normal skin.

- Keep your fingernails as short as possible and make them smooth with an Emory board. This will reduce the chances that an accidental scratch will damage the skin.

- Use sedating antihistamines sparingly but wisely to reduce itching, especially in your sleep. Believe it or not, you can and do scratch in your sleep and this can result in injury to your skin.

- Buy some sunscreen and use it regularly so you avoid sunburn. Try not to get tanned or sunburn as this dries out your skin. Remember to buy sunscreen that has an SPF of 15 or more. There are special sunscreens for the face that can be used all over the skin and is felt to be less irritating than regular sunscreen.

- If you swim in a swimming pool, there is bromine or chlorine in those pools that can be very irritating to people with eczema. Make every effort to take a shower immediately after swimming and use a mild cleanser on your entire body before applying a head to toe moisturizer.

Practice the "Soak and Seal" Technique

There are a lot of things out there that make your skin drier. These include being in windy places, living in low humidity, using specific soaps, using skin care products that contain alcohol and washing your body without applying the right kind of moisturizer afterword.

The first step is to put water back into your skin. This involves taking at least one shower or bath per day using warm but not hot water for at least 10-15 minutes. Make sure you don't scrub your skin with a washcloth and that you use a gentle cleansing wash or bar soap.

When you have finished the bath, pat (do not rub) the water away from the skin and then immediately use the medicine cream or moisturizer to the skin. Try to do it within 3 minutes of getting out of the shower or bath in order to seal in the water. Don't apply moisturizer over the top of creams used as medicines for eczema.

Moisturizers and Cleansers to Use

Your doctor may recommend a specific cleanser and moisturizer to use. Feel free to use moisturizer whenever your skin becomes dry or feels itchy. You'll need a lot so buy the biggest container possible once you know it works as it will save you money.

There are many skin cleansers to choose from. Select one that is designed for people who have sensitive skin. Some specifically gentle cleansers are:

- Basis®
- Oil of Olay®
- Dove®
- Eucerin®

- Aveeno®
- Oilatum®
- Neutrogena®

The next component to keeping your skin moist is to use excellent moisturizers. Remember that creams and ointments are much preferable over lotions that contain drying amounts of alcohol in them. Some good moisturizing agents include:

- Eucerin® Cream
- Aquaphor® Ointment
- Cetaphil® Cream
- Vanicream®

If your eczema involves having a red or itchy scalp, consider a coal tar shampoo, such as T-Gel®. Other helpful shampoos include T-Sal® and Head and Shoulders® shampoo.

Avoid Things That Make Eczema Worse

There are a lot of things you can do that can make your eczema worse. One is the itch-scratch cycle noted above. Another is chemical irritants, including detergents as mentioned above. Other irritants include the use of certain fragrances and soaps that irritate the skin and cause you to itch. Keep the temperature of the area you're in cool and the humidity level high. Use a humidifier year round if you have to. Even if it's winter, wear cool, loose fitting clothing to maximize air flow to the skin.

Consider seeing an allergist to determine if any things are causing you to have an allergic form of eczema. Possible allergens include furry animal dander, feathered animal droppings, dust mites, mold, pollens, chemicals, metals and foods. The doctor will do blood testing, skin testing or patch tests to see if you have a reaction to an item in your lifestyle. There are usually measures you can take to avoid the allergen you find yourself allergic to.

Stress Reduction

Eczema is strongly related to your emotions and stress level. When you're under stress, you tend to scratch more and this brings on the itch-scratch cycle. You can have a bad case of eczema from a pile up of day-to-day stressors or from one big stressor.

Some helpful things you can do is to learn about eczema as much as possible by reading this guide, have family members and friends support you as much as possible, learn relaxation skills and coping skills, and get help for dealing with stress and emotional distress if you believe you need it.

Have an Action Plan

Having an action plan means that you know what to do when your eczema is mild, moderate and severe. Know when to see the doctor and know what to do when your eczema is too severe for you to manage.

Recognize When You Have an Infection

People with eczema frequently have their skin barrier compromised or damaged. This means they are more prone to infection. If you have eczema, you should know the signs and symptoms of a skin infection because it is likely you will get an infection sometime during your lifetime. These signs and symptoms include:

- Having pus-filled bumps or bumps oozing fluid

- Having increased redness
- Having honey colored scabs or crusti-ness.
- You have fever blisters or cold sores

Talk to your doctor immediately if you see any of these things on your skin so you can be treated with an antibiotic.

Chapter 5: Treating Eczema with Natural Supplements and Vital Nutrients

It turns out that different types of eczemas are caused by different nutrient deficiencies. Not knowing which nutrient deficiency is causing your eczema means a missed chance to cure a disease that is most annoying. It is often said that eczema can't be cured. The exception is an eczema caused by a nutrient deficiency. Having the right nutrients in your body could mean the difference between itching and not itching.

When you see the doctor for eczema, most likely you will get a prescription for cortisone cream or some kind of oral steroid to block inflammation. While this will help control your rash, it won't actually cure the disease. It usually comes back when the corticosteroid is stopped. It doesn't really cure the disease.

You can have two possible types of eczema: contact eczema and atopic dermatitis. If you have contact eczema, you have a reaction to something in direct contact with your skin. It can be a metal, like nickel or lead; it can be a solvent like acetone, which is particularly drying also to the skin. Cosmetics can cause contact dermatitis.

If it's not contact dermatitis, then nutrients play a big role in the development of the dermatitis. This is when it pays to know what nutrients are necessary for the skin. The skin is, of course, the biggest organ of the body and it needs its own set of nutrients for proper health. A skin low in nutrients is usually a skin with eczema. For this reason, you need proper nutrition and extra nutrients to keep your skin healthy.

Let's take a look at the nutrients necessary for good skin health. If you have eczema, you can have a deficiency of any one or more of these nutrients:

- **Vitamin A**. Vitamin A is an especially important nutrient for skin health. Vitamin A is found within carotenoids, substances often found with yellow and green fruits and veggies. The fruits and vegetables most likely to cure eczema are cantaloupe, peaches, carrots, yellow squash, pumpkin, beet greens, asparagus, collard greens, broccoli, kale, spinach, turnip greens, Swiss chard, and watercress. Non-vegetable sources of vitamin A include fish liver oil and fish liver.

- **Essential Fatty Acids** (EFA). These are so important to well-fed skin. You can get essential fatty acids from seed oils that have been mechanically pressed from the seeds without using solvents in the process. They include hemp seed oil, flaxseed oil and pumpkin seed oil. Because these are oils that are sensitive to light, heat and oxygen, make sure you buy a little at a time so that they don't sit on the shelf for long periods. Try drinking a tablespoon of seed oil per day, plain or mixed with juice.

Omega-3 fatty acids come primarily from fish. In one double blind study, patients received 1.8 grams of omega 3 fatty acids had reductions in scaling, itching and severity of eczema compared to those that just received olive oil. Omega 6 fatty acids are found in evening primrose oil. This was found to be much better than placebo when treating the itching of eczema.

- **Vitamin B Complex**. People with eczema tend to get a great deal better when they take a B complex vitamin. This is a vitamin that is actually a cluster of B vitamins that are supposed to be taken together. That's how they work—together. For example, biotin is one of the B vitamins. If you take it without any of the other B vitamins, you can actually trigger deficiencies of the other B vitamins. So talk to a reputable health food store about which are the best B complex vitamins to take and take them at least two to three times per week.

- **Topical Vitamin E**. Mix vitamin E oil with lavender essential oil as a way to soothe skin afflicted with eczema. Vitamin E can be cut out of caplets that contain the oil. It nourishes the skin from the outside. Know that it takes several months to grow normal skin cells so keep up the process for at least that long.

- **Vitamin C**. This vitamin has been studied by researchers and has been found to be helpful in the treatment of eczema. In one randomized, crossover, double blind study on severely affected eczema patients ages 3-21, vitamin C given at 50-75 mg/kg slow release supplementation, helped eczema patients after about 6 months of therapy. Those patients who received vitamin C needed half as many courses of antibiotics from infections due to eczema. It is believed, too, that vitamin C had a positive effect on the immune system, in particular, neutrophil chemotaxis and lymphocyte activity. A better immune system means that eczema can be counteracted.

- **Selenium**. Some people with eczema have low levels of glutathione peroxidase, which is a selenium-containing enzyme. This points to the distinct possibility that selenium is necessary for healthy skin. One open trial of selenium found that if one has low levels of glutathione peroxidase, the skin wasn't healthy. Skin got better when selenium increased the glutathione peroxidase levels. Another study looked at giving the combination of selenium and vitamin E with good results.

- **Sodium Restriction**. The levels of sweat sodium (salt) are high in patients who have atopic eczema. One very old study from 1912 indicated that salt restriction was a good idea in eczema patients. This was especially so in patients who had a secretory aspect in their rash. Within 3-4 days, itching was less and after about 3 weeks, the rashes were improved in appearance. It may be a good idea to reduce sodium in your diet and see if your eczema improves.

- **Zinc**. There appears to be a sub-group of people with eczema who don't have enough zinc in their system. Worse lesions are associated with lowest zinc levels and skin infections are probable. Copper levels, on the other hand, seem to be high in hair samples of children and adults with eczema. High copper levels lower the absorption of zinc so having too much copper causes a reduction in zinc. It is suggested that you take 50 mg of zinc chelate three times daily with remission of the eczema after 3-8 months.

If you think that your eczema is caused by a nutrient deficiency, seek the advice of a nutritionist or a doctor who specializes in nutrient deficiencies. As you have seen, there are a variety of nutrients that can be lacking when you have eczema. It may take months of trying one nutrient after another until you find one that works.

If you are taking a supplement and it seems to help the itching after a week or two, it is likely that it will continue over several months toward actual healing of the eczema lesions. In fact, it may take a year or so before the right combination of nutrients is finally discovered in your situation.

Chapter 6: Natural Remedies To Treat Eczema

Herbal Remedies

Long before doctors had prednisone and corticosteroid cream, there were healthcare practitioners that provided perfectly acceptable herbal remedies and homeopathic remedies for eczema. In fact, herbal remedies have enjoyed centuries of success in treating this condition. Herbal remedies take away the inflammation found in the skin and help manage the immune response. Herbal remedies for eczema include:

- **Green Tea**. Green tea has good antioxidant and anti-inflammatory properties and can be applied to the skin or perhaps drunk at one cup twice to three times per day. Remember that it takes many months to see healthy skin show up.

- **Chamomile and Thyme Oils**. These are used together to soothe eczema topically, particularly when used for the treatment of eczema in children.

- **Rehmannia Root (unprocessed), Red Peony Root, Moutan Root Bark and Scrophularia Root**. These roots and barks work together to cleanse the blood of toxic agents. It improves the function of the liver that also gets rid of blood toxins. The end result is detoxification of the skin.

- **Lonicera Flower Buds and Forsythia fruit**. These can help the lungs get rid of toxins so that the skin has fewer toxins to deal with. It is commonly used in Traditional Chinese Medicine.

- **Scute Root, Phellodendron Stem Bark, Gardenia fruit**. These are used together to cleanse the body entirely, including the lungs, liver, stomach, intestines and kidneys. It causes a reduction in skin inflammation caused by eczema or atopic dermatitis.

- **Cicada slough, Fraxinella root and Kochia fruit**. These herbal remedies help to expel toxic substances from the skin so that itching and redness of the skin found in atopic dermatitis or eczema.

- **Atractylodes Rhizome and White Atractylodes Rhizome**. These herbal substances help improve the function of the immune system and can strengthen the way the skin's protective system reacts to attacks by allergens.

- **Salvia Root and Salvia Rhizome**. This improves the blood supply and the circulation of the blood. The end result is better nourishment of the cells of the skin.

- **Herbal extract of Licorice Gel**. This gel has been found in a double blind study to reduce the swelling, redness and itching when used as a 2 percent gel.

- **Chamomile cream**. This was compared to 0.5 percent hydrocortisone cream and was found to be better than the hydrocortisone cream in the management of eczema. The study, however, was not double blinded.

- **Evening Primrose oil and Borage Oil.** These oils contain gamma linolenic acid or GLA, which has been known to correct deficiencies in essential fatty acids. These oils are helpful in the management of eczema and can be used orally or topically.

Other Natural Remedies

Believe it or not, **probiotics** have been found to change the course of eczema. Probiotics are healthy bacteria that take the place of bad bacteria in the colon. Your immune system is improved and your digestive system is able to act as a better barrier to toxins and other agents that can contribute to eczema.

There have been recent studies showing that infants who get eczema have a different set of intestinal bacteria when compared to babies that don't have these bacteria in their system. It is believed that if pregnant women take probiotics, they will inadvertently colonize their babies with the healthy bacteria, thus reducing eczema.

One study on more than 1200 women had some of them take the probiotic agent 2-4 weeks before delivery. The study found that, at birth, the infants had the same bacterial milieu as their mothers. Those with a healthy probiotic profile also had a reduced incidence of eczema. The eczema prevention lasted for up to two years in these infants. Probiotics have also been used in the treatment of eczema in children that already had eczema. Probiotics can prevent symptoms of food allergies in those children who are already sensitized.

One of the most commonly used strains used to protect people from eczema is Lactobacillus GG. In addition Lactobacillus fermentum, Lactobacillus reuteri, Lactobacillus rhamnosus and Bifidobacteria lactis have been found to be effective, especially when taken along with the prebiotic agent called galacto oligosaccharides.

Seek a medical opinion before using probiotics to treat your eczema. When giving probiotics to kids, make sure they have a good immune system. If they don't, then taking a probiotic agent or agents is probably not a good idea.

Homeopathy and Eczema

Practitioners of homeopathy have several remedies for eczema patients. If you have eczema and would like to do homeopathy, seek the advice of a good practitioner in the field so that you get the specific remedy for your condition. Some choices of homeopathic treatments include the following agents:

- **Antimonium crudum**. This is an agent that seems to work best with patients who have eczema that is thick with cracked skin along with indigestion. These are people who tend to be more sensitive than others and are more sentimental than others. They crave things like vinegar and vinegar pickles and can be overweight from these cravings. Kids who need this treatment are often irritable and shy; they have worsened itching when exposed to sun or when too warm. This remedy is great for eczema, impetigo, warts and calluses.

- **Arsenicum album**. This is a remedy best used for people who have eczema and who are restless, compulsive, orderly and anxious. They have intensely burning and itching skin that is made much worse by scratching. Heat actually makes the eczema symptoms better. Indigestion in these people is common and they often feel chilly until they are treated with Arsenicum album.

- **Arum triphyllum**. This is a remedy that works best with eczema that occurs around the mouth or face. The individual often has eczema of the chin with cracked lips that are raw from picking the affected area. There can be added symptoms of hoarseness and throat irritation.

- **Calcarea carbonica**. This remedy works best with eczema patients who also have clammy feet and hands. Their eczema is worse in the winter season and these people are often tired with any exertion. They feel anxious and ill when working too hard. They often crave sweets or possibly eggs, have a slow metabolism and weight issues.

- **Calendula**. This is a great remedy in homeopathic form when you have eczematous skin that easily gets infected.

It can be used topically in gel form, lotion form or as a tincture. It soothes skin that is irritated from having eczema. Inflammation is reduced but not specifically suppressed when using these topical agents.

- **Graphites**. This homeopathic remedy is especially good for those with leathery and tough skin from eczema or other skin disorders. Places most often affected by this type of eczema are the skin behind the ears, the hands, or around the mouth. There is often golden crusting of the skin. The eczema itching is worse when the patient is warm and itching can often cause bleeding of the skin. These are people who have difficulty with morning concentration.

- **Hepar sulphuris calcareum**. People who do well with this remedy tend to be extremely sensitive and are often cold. Their eczema is painful and becomes easily infected. The hands and feet are often affected and do not heal easily. This is a person who is really irritable and vulnerable. They have low resistances to infection and illness.

- **Mezereum**. This remedy for eczema is reserved for people who have a great deal of anxiety and a nervous stomach. These people get strong eruptions that start out like blisters and form thick crusts and oozing. The skin gets thick from chronic itching. The application of cold makes the itching better. These are people who crave fat and like the open air.

- **Rhus Toxicodendron**. The person who best uses this remedy has blistery eczema, severe itching and eczema that gets better with the application of heat. The individual is uncomfortable, which makes them restless and is often irritable and very anxious. Other symptoms include stiffness of the muscles and a craving for milk. Gentle motion and warmth helps the muscle stiffness.

- **Petrolatum**. This is a remedy that works best for people who have eczema that is thick and dry, often cracked. The fingertips and palms are mostly affected and winter makes the eczema worse. The person feels a cold sensation to the skin after scratching it too much. Itching feels worse at night when the person gets into a warm bed. Infections of the skin are common with this kind of eczema.

- **Sulphur**. People who have eczema that is burning, inflamed and itchy do better with this remedy. The areas affected are often red, crusty and scaling with either dry or moist eruptions. It tends to work well with people who have used other medications for their eczema unsuccessfully.

Dosing Homeopathy Remedies

Let the homeopathy provider select the specific dosage according to your symptoms. The higher the dilution, the higher is the strength of the remedy. Often, homeopathic providers have you take one dose and wait to see if there is a response. If there is a visible improvement, you'll stay on the same dosage and let the eczema heal. If not, the dosage can be improved until a response is reached.

Chapter 7: Treating Children with Eczema

It's a sad fact that many sufferers from this itchy condition are children. Babies have eczema as well and can't usually scratch what itches them. And yet, many of the stronger treatments out there for eczema can't be used in children.

In children, the main symptom is a red, itchy rash. Sometimes the rash can be oozing and scaly and can begin sometime in infancy up to about five years of age. It is a rash that is basically incurable and will come and go. Doctors can diagnose eczema just by looking at the rash and finding a typical rash especially in the creases of the elbows, knees and ankles in older children and on the cheeks, arms and legs in infants.

Preventing Eczema in Children

The trick to dealing with eczema in children is preventing flare ups of the disease. This means no bubble baths, no harsh soaps, cleaning the house of dust mites and avoiding any situation that overheats your child and stops sweating. Put your child in cotton or cotton blend clothing and don't have them wear wool or polyester clothes.

You should bathe your child daily with bathwater that is lukewarm. Use a moisturizing and gentle soap and rinse it off well. Immediately after bathing, use a cream or ointment on their skin that will seal in the moisture you just put in during the bathing process. The greasier the ointment, the better will it be at keeping moisture in the child's skin. Make sure you apply moisturizer at least two to three times daily.

There are prescription creams that don't contain any steroids that can be used in place of a regular moisturizer. Some of them are Atopiclair, Mimyx and Hylira. Ask your doctor if your child is a candidate for any of these creams.

Treating Eczema Flare-ups

Common treatments for flare-ups of eczema are topical over the counter steroid creams and a few non-steroidal creams such as Elidel (pimecrolimus) and Protopic (tacrolimus) creams. These can't be used in kids under 2 nor can they be used for a long period of time. Topical steroid creams are generally very mild, even in children and they can be used in any body area, including the face. Stronger steroid creams can be gotten with a prescription but must be used sparingly and not on the face. Very strong steroid creams are avoided in children.

Commonly used prescription-strength steroid creams include:

- Dermatop®
- Elocon®
- Cutivate®
- Locoid Lipocream®
- 0.1 percent triamcinolone cream

While side effects like stretch marks and thinning skin can still occur with these creams, they are far better when used sparingly than the super strong creams. None of them should be used on the face.

There are Immunomodulators or steroid-free medications for kids, like Protopic and Elidel that are used twice daily for kids over the age of two. They can be used on the face to prevent flare-ups of the disease. Put them on at the first sign of itching.

Kids can always use antihistamines to treat the itching of eczema. Because they are sedating, medications like Benadryl® and Atarax® can be used to control nighttime itching. If there is daytime itching, you can use cold compresses on the affected area.

Eczema Facts

While eczema is not curable, many children outgrow the condition or have an improvement as they get older. Eczema does run in families so you may have more than one child affected with the disease. Put the moisturizing cream or ointment over the top of the medicated creams and not the other way around. Baths are truly to be taken daily for around 10 minutes at a time with ointment or cream applied less than 3 minutes after the bath so that the skin stays as moisturized as possible.

Remember that winter exacerbates eczema so be prepared with extra moisturizer. Swimming season is another time when extra vigilance needs to happen regarding using moisturizer. Skin infections are always possible so have Neosporin® on hand for these kinds of situations. If you can't seem to control your child's eczema at home, make use of a pediatric dermatologist who can help with prescription strength medications and other ideas.

Chapter 8: Recipes of Easy-to-make Meals That Give You Eczema Relief

We've already talked about the importance of good nutrition and healthy nutrients in the management of eczema. Even knowing all of this, however, it is sometimes hard to put together meals that you can just throw together that will manage the disease. The purpose of this chapter is to give you some ideas of meals and recipes that will make you your skin as itch-free as possible.

We will also keep in mind, as much as possible, the fact that many people with eczema have allergies to certain foods. There are things you can do to make substitutions if necessary so that you're cooking with things that don't make eczema worse.

Breakfast

Breakfast should focus on protein meals like eggs and bacon, eggs and any other meat plus fruits, cooked or raw. If you think you have a problem with gluten, you need to avoid bread, such as toast, muffins or other bread-like items. You should also be wary of cow's milk such as cow's milk with cereal. Try juice or water if you are thirsty.

Lunch and Dinner Recipes

These are some recipes you might want to try for either lunch or dinner that are designed with few things that will make your eczema worse. Try them!

Avocado and Quinoa Salad

Quinoa is good for eczema because it is free of gluten. It is about 18 percent protein, containing 9 essential fatty acids, low sodium content and high fiber. It is rich in B vitamins, vitamin E, Manganese, iron, magnesium, copper and phosphorus. Avocado is great for the nutrition of your skin because it contains the essential fatty acids your skin needs. Serves 4.

Ingredients:

- 1 c red quinoa
- 2 avocados (cut up)
- 2 basil leaves (fresh)
- Dried tomatoes (a few)
- One onion (green)

For the dressing:

- Lemon juice (using 2 lemons)
- 1/4 c olive oil
- 1 minced garlic clove
- Salt
- Pinch of cayenne pepper

Directions:

Rinse off quinoa in cool water and allow to drain. Using a saucepan, boil salt and 2 c water. Put in quinoa. Cover pot and reduce the heat so it simmers. Cook about 20 minutes. When quinoa has healed, mix the ingredients together and toss with the dressing. If you have parsley, use it as a garnish.

Endive and Crab Salad

Endive is nicely low in calories and contains great stores of vitamins C and A. It has plenty of fiber in it as well. Crab has selenium in it, which acts as an antioxidant and chromium, which is great for your cholesterol. The cayenne pepper in it helps your blood circulation. Serves 5.

Ingredients:

- 1 pound cooked crab
- 5 heads of Belgian Endive separated into spears
- 2 tbsp yogurt (plain)
- 1 tsp lemon juice
- 1/2 tsp salt
- 1/4 tsp cayenne pepper
- 1 bunch chopped fresh chives

Directions:

In a bowl, mix ingredients together, including chunked crab. Pour this mixture over the endive spears and garnish with chopped chives.

Fennel Salad

Fennel is good for you because it contains quercetin, a flavonoid antioxidant. It also contains great amounts of vitamin C. Serves 4.

Ingredients:

- 1 finely chopped fennel bulb
- 2 tablespoons fresh lemon juice
- 2 tablespoons extra virgin olive oil
- 1 clove minced garlic
- Parsley or cilantro

Directions:

Cut up all ingredients and toss together, garnishing with cilantro or parsley.

Chicken Salad

Because this is made of chicken, it doesn't inflame your skin as much as beef might. Try this during the winter season because it will give you plenty of nutrients. If you can get a hold of organic chicken and organic vegetables, use these. Serves 4.

Ingredients:

- 4 pieces of chicken
- 4 carrots
- 2 leeks
- 2 sticks chopped celery
- 2 cloves garlic
- 2 onions, finely chopped
- 1 turnip
- 1 bay leaf
- 1/2 cup lemon juice
- Olive oil
- Salt to taste
- Pepper to taste
- 1 c vegetable broth
- 1/2-1 quart water

Directions:

Brown the onions and half of the veggies along with 2 tbsp of olive oil in a sauce pan.

Then add the chicken to this mixture followed by the rest of the vegetables, salt and pepper. Add broth and water. Add lemon juice. Do not cover but instead cook for 45 minutes. On plate, put chicken piece on and cover with sauce and veggies. Mix sauce with a bit of cream and 2 egg yolks for a thicker sauce.

Salmon with Apples

Salmon is good for you with eczema because it is a great source of omega 3 fatty acids. Make sure the salmon you use is the freshest possible. Serves 4.

Ingredients:

- One pound thinly sliced salmon fillets
- Slices from one apple
- Juice from 2 lemons
- 8 tbsp extra virgin olive oil
- 2 tbsp chopped shallots
- 1 tbsp chopped fresh dill
- 1 tbsp chopped basil
- 1 minced clove of garlic
- Salt and pepper to taste
- Capers as a garnish

Directions:

Arrange the salmon slices on a large serving dish. Place apple slices on top. Make the dressing out of the olive oil, lemons, herbs and salt and pepper. Pour the dressing on the salmon and marinate for 20 minutes before adding capers and serving.

Ginger and Carrot Soup

Carrots are great for you because it has no saturated fat, no cholesterol, and plenty of vitamin C, fiber, vitamin A, vitamin K, potassium, niacin, thiamin, folate, manganese and vitamin B6. The butternut squash is high in beta carotene, which is an excellent antioxidant that cuts down on inflammation. Expect to find vitamin C, folate, fiber, potassium, manganese, vitamin B complex, copper and omega 3 fatty acids in the butternut squash. Serves 4.

Ingredients:

- 1/2 of a butternut squash
- 1 pound diced carrots
- 1 diced onion
- 1 c orange juice
- 2 tbsp vegetable oil
- 2 cloves minced garlic
- 1 piece sliced ginger
- 3 c water
- Cinnamon to taste
- Salt to taste
- Pepper to taste

Directions:

Heat oven to 375 degrees. Place scooped out squash with the cut side up in a baking sheet covered with foil. Bake this for 45 minutes or until squash is soft. In a large saucepan, heat olive oil and cook onion and garlic. Add water, diced squash carrots and ginger pieces. Boil for up to 20 minutes or until ingredients are soft. Puree the mixture until smooth. Add boiling water to thin the soup if necessary. Add orange juice and spices, heating the soup to the proper temperature.

Vegetarian Stir Fry

You can choose different vegetables in this stir fry depending on the seasons. The selection in the recipe has many nutrients that are good for the management of eczema. Serves 4.

Ingredients:

- Cut up broccoli
- 2 sliced large onions
- 1/2 c snow peas
- Cut up baby bok choy
- Thinly cut carrots-2
- 2 cloves minced garlic
- Red or yellow bell peppers cut up
- 1 tbsp soy sauce
- 1/4 c olive oil
- 1 c water

Directions:

In a large pot, put in water and boil it. Add all vegetables except bok choy. Cover this pot and cook for around 7 minutes. Drain veggies and put it in the pan along with the bok choy. Add garlic, soy sauce and oil to the vegetables. Cook together for about 5 minutes. Serve over cooked brown rice if desired.

Zucchini Pie

Zucchini is high in vitamins C and A; it is low in calories. The soya cream is used in place of crème fraiche. It is better for you as well.

Ingredients:

- 6 eggs
- 8 zucchini
- 1/2 pound of soya crème
- 2 tsp olive oil
- A bunch of chervil
- A bunch of fresh mint
- A bunch of parsley

For tomato sauce:

- 1/4 c olive oil
- 2 minced green peppers
- 6 chopped tomatoes
- 4 minced cloves of garlic
- 3 minced onions
- Salt and pepper to taste

Directions:

Thinly slice the zucchini. Heat up the olive oil in a large saucepan. Cook the zucchini for about 4-5 minutes. Drain the zucchini and set aside. Mix the crème, herbs, eggs, salt and pepper Mix the zucchini and liquid egg mixture together in a baking dish. Bake this mixture for 40 minutes. In the meantime, Heat tomatoes over medium heat with oil and add garlic, onions and green peppers until cooked. Put this sauce in the refrigerator. Then cut up egg/zucchini pie and put sauce over it.

Almond Sesame Cakes

Both almonds and sesame seeds have loads of essential fatty acids, which are healthy for your skin. When you eat almonds, you also have a good source of magnesium, vitamin E, calcium, and flavonoids. These are little desserts that are actually healthy for you. Share them as eating them all means you're getting too much sugar. Makes 10 little cakes.

Ingredients:

- 3 eggs
- 1/2 pound almond powder
- 120 g brown sugar
- 3 tsp sesame seeds
- 40 g Tahini
- 2 tsp almond or orange extract

Directions:

Preheat oven to 200 degrees. Mix eggs, Tahini, extract, and sugar together and then add the almond powder. Mix well. Put in 8 x8 pan and sprinkle with sesame seeds. Bake for 45 minutes. Cut into ten rectangular pieces.

Eggplant and Zucchini

This recipe is good for eczema because it contains many vitamins and minerals. It is gluten free and dairy free. Serves 4.

Ingredients:

- 2 zucchini
- 2 eggplants
- 2 cloves garlic, minced
- 1 shallot
- 1 tbsp olive oil
- Salt to taste
- Pepper to taste

Directions:

Cut up the eggplant into 1/2 inch slices. Boil eggplant pieces in water for about ten minutes. You can cook it in a slow cooker or pressure cooker, too. Drain it well. Mix the olive oil, minced garlic, salt, and pepper as a marinade. In a big bowl, place eggplant and zucchini together in layers and add marinade to mix. Marinate for at least 12 hours in the refrigerator before serving.

Greek Appetizer

This Greek appetizer can fight Candida and contains acidophilus that acts as an excellent probiotic. Garlic fights fungus as well as does olive oil. Replace yogurt with goat yogurt if you are intolerant of lactose. Serves 4.

Ingredients:

- 2 c yogurt (plain)
- 3 cloves minced garlic
- 1 cucumber, peeled, de-seeded and grated
- 1/4 c olive oil
- 1 tsp basil
- 1 tbsp lemon juice
- 1/2 tsp dill
- Sea salt to taste

Directions:

Put cucumber in a strainer and lightly salt it. Let it sit like this for 15 minutes to draw out the water. Drain. Then mix the rest of the ingredients together. Cover and refrigerate for half an hour before serving.

Veggie Burgers

These veggie burgers get their texture from mushrooms so that meat isn't necessary. You get your selenium, phosphorus, magnesium and potassium from these mushrooms. They contain antioxidants that are healthy for your skin. Serves 4.

Ingredients:

- 2 eggs
- 1 c garbanzo beans, cooked, drained
- 1 clove minced garlic
- 2 c chopped fresh mushrooms
- 1 med chopped onion
- 1/4 c wheat germ
- Salt
- Cayenne pepper
- 1 bunch fresh cilantro

Directions:

Sautee onion in olive oil for four minutes or until onions are tender. Add mushrooms and garlic. Cook for about 5 minutes. Set this mixture aside for a little bit and mash the garbanzo beans with fork. Add everything but the wheat germ and mix together. Let it sit for a few minutes and form into four burgers. Roll burgers in wheat germ and cook in pan with olive oil—about three minutes per side. Serve on buns or on their own with condiments.

Sugar free Nut Snacks

These snack cakes are sugar free, which is good for those with yeast problems. There is no dairy or gluten in this snack and they still taste great! Nuts themselves are rich in essential fatty acids and have other good nutrients in them. Eat a few of them every day but not peanuts. Makes 14 cakes.

Ingredients:

- 2 eggs
- 2 c brown rice flour
- 5 tsp baking powder
- 1 tbsp oats
- A mixture of sesame seeds, pumpkin seeds, flax seeds, sunflower seeds, etc.
- 1/2 tsp salt
- 2 tbsp olive oil
- 1/4 c water

For topping:

- 1 almond or walnut
- Coarse sea salt
- Dried herbs—whatever taste good to you

Directions:

Mix dry ingredients all together. Add eggs and olive oil. Add water to make a sticky, smooth dough. Knead the dough a little bit and then make fourteen small buns out of it. Add nut to top and sprinkle with herbs and salt while the dough balls are sitting on a greased cookie tin. Place in the oven and bake at 360 degrees for approximately 30 minutes or until a knife embedded in one of them comes out clean.

Zucchini Soup

This is a soup for the summertime and is a soup rich in vitamin C and vitamin A, both of which are healthy for your skin. This is a great chilled soup! Serves 4.

Ingredients:

- 700 grams or 1.5 pounds of diced, un-peeled organic zucchini
- 2 egg yolks
- 3 minced onions
- The juice of one lemon
- 1 teaspoon each of fresh chives, mint and coriander
- 9 tablespoons olive oil
- 1 can vegetable broth
- Salt to taste
- Pepper to taste

Directions:

Mix the vegetable broth with 3/4 quart hot water. In another cooking pot, place 2 tbsp of the olive oil and then add onion, allowing it to sauté until cooked through. Add the diced zucchini, pepper and salt. Add the broth to the pot and allow to boil. Reduce heat and allow mixture to simmer for at least 20 minutes. Mix lemon juice with egg yolks and with the re-mainder of the olive oil. When all is cooked, puree the soup in a food processor and add egg mixture while still mixing soup. Adjust seasonings and cover with saran wrap. Chill the soup in the refrigerator for at least 4 hours. Serve the soup chilled with coriander mint and chives. It actually tastes best when made the day before eating.

Garlic Sweet Potatoes

This is a side dish recipe that has anti-inflammatory properties. Sweet potatoes contain a great amount of beta carotene, which is a type of vitamin A. It also contains a lot of vitamin C. Sweet potatoes are considered healing for the skin because of its antioxidant properties. The garlic, turmeric and olive oil have many anti-inflammatory properties. Serves 4.

Ingredients:

- 1 large sweet potato
- 1/2 tsp turmeric
- 2 tbsp olive oil
- 4 garlic cloves, minced
- 1-2 tsp fresh, minced parsley

Directions:

Heat a tablespoon of olive oil in pan so you can lightly sauté the garlic. Set the garlic aside. Then sauté the cut up potatoes and turmeric in the rest of the olive oil until potatoes are browned. Add the garlic back to the sweet potatoes and garnish with parsley.

Summery Strawberry Sorbet

This is the greatest sorbet when used with fresh, sweet strawberries. Use it as a great dessert or to cleanse your palate between different courses of your meal. Strawberries contain vitamin C and also have good anti-inflammatory and antioxidant properties. While sorbet is healthy and without dairy products, the sugar content means that you shouldn't eat it very often. It is a perfect dessert for people who happen to be lactose intolerant. Serves 6.

Ingredients:

- One pound of strawberries or a pound of frozen strawberries without sugar
- 1 tablespoon lemon juice
- 1/4 pound sugar
- 1/2 quart water

Directions:

Dissolve the sugar in the water over low heat until sugar is completely dissolved. Let the mixture boil for a minute and set aside. Clean and wash strawberries removing their stems. Grind strawberries into food mill, extracting the seeds until the puree is seedless.

Add sugar and lemon juice to the strawberry mixture so all is mixed. Put the mixture in an 8 x 8 pan that is stainless steel. Cover with saran wrap and freeze for 2-3 hours in a freezer. Let stand on the countertop so it thaws a little bit before serving. Use mint to garnish the sorbet.

Ginger Tofu

This involves grilling tofu as an entrée. You can serve it alongside sautéed vegetables. If you squeeze lemon juice on the tofu before serving, it tastes even better! Serves 4.

Ingredients:

- 1 pound extra firm tofu, sliced into 1/2 inch slices
- 1/2 tbsp garlic, minced
- 1 tbsp fresh ginger, minced
- 1 tbsp sesame oil
- 1/2 tbsp curcumin
- Soy sauce

Directions:

First drain tofu and then slice it. Wrap it in paper towels and press gently on them to dry them out. Heat up the sesame oil in a saucepan to medium. Stir in ginger, curcumin and garlic for a minute and then add tofu, grilling them until browned. This is about a five minute job. Sprinkle with soy sauce before grilling them, five minutes per side. Serve right away.

Pesto with Pine Nuts

The pesto itself keeps in the refrigerator for a week. It can be sealed and frozen for a few months. The recipe is nondairy and has anti-bacterial and anti-inflammatory properties. It also contains a great deal of iron, calcium and vitamins. Essential fatty acids are found in the olive oil and the pine nuts are rich in protein and in monounsaturated fats. Serve this on pasta or on cooked vegetables. Serves 4.

Ingredients:

- 40 grams of pine nuts
- 4 cloves minced garlic
- 2 c packed fresh basil leaves
- 1/2 c olive oil
- Salt to taste
- Pepper to taste

Directions:

Using a blender or food processor, chop the basil leaves. It may take many small batches to accomplish the blending. Add half the pine nuts along with garlic salt and pepper. Blend the mixture. Brown half of the pine nuts and blend. Then slowly blend in the olive oil until a thick paste forms. Add more olive oil if necessary. Toss the mixture with veggies or pasta.

Mexican Rice

This is a great recipe to make Mexican rice yourself. It is gluten free and dairy free and helps stabilize blood sugar levels. It is high in vitamin B1 and is anti-inflammatory when mixed with vegetables. Serves 6.

Ingredients:

- 1 c white rice
- 1/2 finely chopped green pepper
- 1 tbsp vegetable oil
- 1/2 white onion, chopped finely
- 1.5 c chicken broth
- 1 jalapeno pepper, chopped
- Chicken bouillon cube
- 1/2 tsp ground cumin
- 1 seeded and chopped tomato
- 1/2 c chopped cilantro
- 1 clove of garlic cut in half
- Salt & pepper to taste

Directions:

Using a medium sauce pan, cook rice in oil for approximately 3 minutes. Pour in chicken broth and allow this to boil. Add green pepper, onion, diced tomato and jalapeno pepper. Add spices and bouillon cube to flavor the rice further. Finally, bring the entire mixture to a boil and cover. Simmer the rice mixture for an additional twenty minutes.

Zucchini Spaghetti

Zucchini is low in calories and are high in ascorbic acid, potassium, folate, zeaxanthin and lutein. As these are heat-sensitive, it is best to eat zucchini that hasn't been cooked too long. Zucchini has great detoxifying and anti-inflammatory effects. Serves 4-6.

Ingredients:

- 24 ounces of zucchini, thinly sliced
- 2 tbsp yeast flakes
- 17 ounces of spaghetti
- 1/2 c walnuts
- Basil leaves 4-5

Directions:

In a frying pan or skillet, heat the oil and add garlic and zucchini. Stir often and cook at higher heat. Zucchinis should be golden brown and crispy outside. Cook pasta and sauté together with zucchini, basil leaves (chopped) and yeast. Serve right away.

Goat Cheese Salad

This contains goat cheese, which is perfect for people who don't tolerate cow's milk cheese. The goat cheese is warm and goes well with the honey. Serves 4.

Ingredients:

- Whole wheat bread—eight slices
- 8 slices of goat cheese
- Lettuce, one head
- Olive oil, 8 teaspoons
- Honey, 8 teaspoons
- Salt & pepper to taste

Directions:

Wash and dry the lettuce, tearing it onto a plate. Season the lettuce with balsamic dressing, salt and pepper. Put a tablespoon of honey on each piece of bread. Put goat's milk cheese on top. Place bread and cheese slices in hot oven until the cheese begins to brown. Serve one slice of bread per plate of lettuce.

Coconut Cake

This is a low fat cake that is butter-free with brown sugar. Makes one cake.

Ingredients:

- 3 eggs
- 150 grams of brown sugar
- 100 grams of coconut
- 150 grams of plain flour
- 1 tsp vanilla sugar
- 250 milliliters of milk
- 1 tsp baking powder

Directions:

Separate the eggs and keep the egg whites aside. Put the yolks in a bowl with the sugar. Mix together and then add flour little by little. Add milk and the rest of the ingredients except the egg whites. Beat the egg whites after putting in a pinch of salt. Fold the ingredients together and pour into 9 x 9 pan. Sprinkle coconut flakes on the mixture as an adornment.

Mushroom Appetizer

This is a salad or an appetizer, depending on how you want to serve it. It is served cold so it is good for summer parties. The small mushrooms used are also called Paris Mushrooms. They are high in fiber and have a great deal of potassium in it. They are also rich in niacin, selenium and riboflavin. The selenium helps vitamin E in cellular protection against oxygen free radicals. Serves 4.

Ingredients:

- 1.2 pounds of white button mushrooms, cleaned and sliced thinly
- 10 tbsp olive oil
- 2 shallots, peeled and sliced
- 3 tbsp cider vinegar
- 1 tbsp basil, fresh and chopped
- 2 tbsp parsley, fresh and chopped
- 1 tbsp coriander, fresh and chopped
- 1 clove garlic, minced
- Salt to taste
- Pepper to taste
- 1 tbsp mustard
- 1 tbsp white wine (optional)

Directions:

Slice mushrooms into a salad bowl and set aside. Make a blend of salt, pepper, wine and vinegar, whisked together. Add mustard to salad dressing and a little bit of olive oil at a time (while whisking). Add herbal ingredients, garlic and shallots. Toss all the ingredients together and refrigerate for up to a half hour before serving in a nice plate or dish.

Apple Mousse

The best apples for this mousse are red delicious. They are healthiest for your skin because of a high collagen and elastin count. They are best eaten raw so you don't lose the nutritional value of the apple. The apples in this recipe are cooked but they still hold good nutritional value along with the honey and yogurt. Serves 4.

Ingredients:

- One pound sweet apples, red or yellow
- 1/2 c yogurt
- 2 tbsp honey
- 2 grams agar

Directions:

Peel, wash and chop up the apples. Place about an inch of water in the bottom of a big pan. Add the apples, agar and honey. Cook on high at first and then over medium heat with the lid on. Cook until the apples grow soft. Mash the apples by hand or with a food processor until you have a smooth puree of apples. Cool this mixture down and whip yogurt. Mix the two ingredients together and pour into four glasses. Allow this mixture to chill before serving. Put sliced almonds and honey atop each glass.

Vegetarian Spanish Rice

This recipe makes use of a rice cooker to make the Spanish rice. Because it is spicy, it could be inflammatory for some patients. Serves 6.

Ingredients:

- One onion, chopped
- 1 c of long grain white rice
- 1/2 of a green pepper, chopped
- 1.5 cups of water
- 1 clove of minced garlic
- 2 tbsp vegetable oil
- 1 cup diced tomatoes including its juice
- 3/4 tsp of cumin
- 2 tsp chili powder
- 1 tsp salt

Directions:

Using a rice cooker, add oil to the basket and turn it on. Heat oil and sauté the onion, green pepper and rice until the rice has become browned. Add the remainder of the ingredients to the rice cooker. Stir it up, cover the cooker and let the cooker cook the rice. You may need to add an additional 1/2 cup of water to the rice mixture if it is too dry.

Avocado Smoothie

This is a smoothie with many good nutritional qualities to it. It provides about twenty essential nutrients like vitamin D, vitamin A, vitamin E and vitamin K. It contains many B vitamins and soluble fiber, which is known to lower cholesterol. The fats it contains are healthy for you and have anti-inflammatory properties. Serves 2.

Ingredients:

- 1 peeled and chopped avocado
- 2 c rice milk or almond milk, unsweetened
- 3 tbsp honey
- 1 tbsp lemon juice
- 5 ice cubes

Directions:

Take all of the ingredients and place them in a blender. Blend until smooth and serve cold.

Almond Pesto Sauce

Ingredients:

- 1 c almonds, blanched
- 2 inch cube of hard Parmesan cheese
- 2 c basil leaves, packed full
- 2 cloves of garlic, minced
- 1/4 c Extra Virgin Olive Oil

Directions:

Process almonds until they are completely finely crumbled. Add garlic and mix. Grate in Parmesan cheese and then add the basil leaves, blending together. While running the food processor, pour in the olive oil slowly. Then add water if the mixture is too thick. Salt the mixture to taste. Store in an air tight container in the refrigerator for up to a week. Serve over pasta, in soups, on baked sweet potatoes or other vegetables.

Smoked Salmon Salad

This is a perfect choice for people who are not allergic to fish. Salmon especially contains essential fatty acids that do a great deal when it comes to controlling eczema. Salmon also has astaxanthin, which is a carotenoid and a good source of vitamin A. The rest of the salad provides a great deal of vitamin C. Serves 2.

Ingredients:

- Romaine lettuce, one small head of organic vegetable
- 4 thinly sliced radishes
- Smoked salmon, 5 ounces, sliced thinly
- 1/2 of a cucumber, peeled and diced
- 2 diced tomatoes
- Juice from 1/2 lemon
- 1 carrot cut diagonally along its length
- 1 tbsp vegetable oil
- 1 tsp fresh ginger root, peeled and minced

Directions:

Wash the romaine lettuce and break into leaves, arranging the leaves on two separate plates. On top of the lettuce, put the salmon, tomatoes and other vegetables. Mix the ginger, vegetable oil and lemon juice by shaking it together in a jar. Pour this over the salad and serve immediately.

Carrot Muffins

These are great because they are gluten free for those who have problems with eczema and gluten. Both the flaxseed and the carrots empower these muffins with anti-inflammatory properties, which fight eczema. Makes a dozen muffins.

Ingredients:

- 1 c rice milk
- An egg
- 1/4 c raisins
- 4 tbsp canola oil
- 2 c quinoa flour
- 1 tsp cinnamon
- 1 tsp guar gum
- 1/4 c brown sugar
- 1 tbsp flaxseed meal
- 1-1/2 tsp baking powder
- 1/2 tsp salt
- 1 c of organic carrots, grated

Directions:

Preheat oven to 400 degrees. Beat rice milk, egg, and canola oil together while you also put the dry ingredients in another bowl. Mix the liquid and solid ingredients together until they have just mixed together (don't over-beat). Fold in the raisins and the carrots. Pour into 12 muffin tins and bake the muffins for 20 minutes. You can use cupcake liners to allow for easier dispensation of the muffins.

Conclusion

Eczema is a chronic skin condition that can affect people of all ages, including infants. It goes by many names, depending on its location and appearance but the most common alternative name is atopic dermatitis.

Eczema is sometimes thought of as an allergic condition but in reality, it is not an allergy but is rather a sensitivity. People with eczema are sensitive to soaps, detergents, wool fabric, animal dander, upper respiratory infections, stress and the mites in house dust. When exposed to these conditions, the skin becomes red, itchy and sometimes scaly with pustules in some cases.

There is no cure for eczema except for limiting exposure to the offending agents and minimizing stress. Besides intense itching, the major negative effects of eczema are its unsightly appearance and the chance of secondary bacterial infection of the skin. Infection can get in excoriated skin that has been scratched too much. For this reason, it is recommended that you keep your nails cut short to minimize damage from scratching.

While eczema can't be cured, it can be treated so that its sufferers aren't miserable. The basic treatment of choice is intense moisturization of the skin. In children who have eczema, for example, it is recommended that you bathe the child every day for 20 minutes in lukewarm water and that moisturizers be applied within three minutes of getting out of the tub and patting the skin dry. The same holds for adults who have this condition.

When moisturizing the skin, ointments and creams are recommended over lotions. Lotions contain alcohol in them, which is inherently drying to the skin. There are a number of recommended creams and ointments, including Aquaphor® and Eucerin®. Aquaphor is an ointment that seals moisture in the skin, while Eucerin® is a cream that basically does the same thing. You can apply moisturizer as much as you want to the areas affected by eczema.

In many cases, moisturizer alone is insufficient to control the itching and the rash. This usually means adding 1 percent hydrocortisone cream to the mix. In many cases this over the counter remedy can relieve the itching. If it doesn't work, a trip to the doctor may be in order. There are stronger corticosteroid creams available by prescription and topical/oral medications that affect the immune system. Many of these medications cannot be used in children and almost all can't be used for long periods of time. There are side effects from all medications used in eczema that can limit treatment.

If you find yourself unable to make use of prescription medication or if you want to try and heal yourself from eczema in a more natural way, you need to understand the interplay of food, nutrients and nutrition with your eczema. Some people suffer from nutrient deficiencies which contribute to their eczema.

The nutrient could be a vitamin, such as vitamin B complex. The nutrient could also be a heavy metal like selenium. You need to replace these nutrients, perhaps one by one, until you see a change in your skin. Eczema doesn't physically change in appearance very quickly so you need to go by the amount of itching you are experiencing and expect healthy skin to begin to be there by 4 months out from the change in nutrients.

The same is true for homeopathic and herbal remedies for eczema. It is the itching and redness that gets better first. This causes the skin to begin to heal and the tough, leathery skin you sometimes see to gradually disappear over several months. There are herbal remedies and homeopathic remedies that have been found to work well with people who have eczema. Some treatments have centuries of positive experiences behind them.

In some cases, what you eat has a great deal to do with getting eczema flare ups or not. For example, some people are gluten-intolerant and others have an allergy to cow's milk (lactose intolerance) that contributes to getting eczema. For this reason, this guide has included an extensive list of recipes that either have anti-inflammatory properties or antioxidant properties. Some contain the same nutrients felt to be lacking in some cases of eczema.

It is possible to live well with eczema if one is careful about what you eat, your stress level and what you usually wear. You should wear cotton or cotton blend clothing that keeps your skin cool and allows it to breathe. If you pay a good deal of attention to moisturizing

the skin and use natural or conventional medications as directed, you can keep your skin
from the adverse effects of the itching and
scratching cycle.

Made in the USA
Monee, IL
06 April 2021

64928947R00075